MW00695966

How To Improve Cellular Health

A Basic Guide To

Cellular Health, Nutrition and Energy

By Jos Struik

Alkmaar

The Netherlands

2019

"If you want to find

the secrets of the universe,

think in terms of

energy, frequency and

vibration."

Nikola Tesla
(1856 – 1943)

Disclaimer

This book is not a medical book and the author is not a medical specialist. The information provided is the author's personal view based on generally available sources. Consult a (medical) specialist if you are in doubt about the impact of this information on your life.

Science and orthodox medicine do not accept the existence of some the methods or treatments mentioned in this book and their possible medical or other relevance, due to a lack of scientific proof in accordance with orthodox medicine standards.

CONTENTS

Introduction

Only in the recent past I learned about "biohacking". I am fortunate enough to be healthy and strong. But I don't take that for granted. It is my mission to share my knowledge and experencies about health at a cellular level with everybody who cares and is open to alternatives. I look for solutions and products that have been proven to be effective. Perhaps not for everybody or in all circumstances. And perhaps not acknowledged by regular or more orthodox medicine. But always based on research and personal findings and shared by others. I focus on health at cellular level, because that's where it all starts. Strengthen your cells and DNA and your body and mind will follow.

According to scientists, health is determined by the conditions of millions of cells composing the body. In order for the body to host life-essential activities such as biochemical reactions and physiological processes, cells need the proper nutrition from vitamins, amino acids, and trace elements. Chronic nutrition deficiency in cells causes cellular dysfunction and renders the whole body vulnerable to various diseases, from minor to serious.

Refilling the cells with the needed nutrients is one way to sustain their bio-energy production and will result in a better health. If, however, the lacking nutrients are not supplemented, the cells' normal functioning is damaged, leading to the opposite: poor health. For the body to function normally and healthily, cells must have nutritional support. Cellular health therefore is based on the foundation of nutrient synergy and regular intake of vitamins and other nutrients essential for good health.

An important function of our cells is to produce the energy our body needs to perform its vital functions. Apart from the right nutrients there are other possibilities to add energy to our body. Since the late 1800's we know that it is also possible to use electrical impulses to improve our energetic health. Through science and new technologies we are now able to work on a wide variety of bodily symptoms, diseases and conditions using energy and frequencies.

In this book I will show how electromedicine, bioresonance and/or frequency therapy can directly improve the cells energy level. These forms of therapy offer a unique, non-invasive, pain-free and natural way of improving one's health and wellbeing. The therapy benefits both physical and mental health by scanning the body, detecting negative frequencies and altering them into healthier ones, to allow cells to complete their tasks without obstructions. There's a growing body of evidence that confirms the benefits of using unique frequency patterns to address various issues, and an increasing number of healthcare providers realize the potential of devices used as part of their therapy.

In the first chapters of this book I will explain what the cell is and how it works. For some that may be a bit too scientific or technical. The bottom line is that each cell plays an important individual role in our body's health. Many diseases start with deficiencies in our cells without us even knowing or feeling it. When we understand the process in our cells and their function, we see why it is vital to pay attention to our cellular health.

In the following chapters I will focus on the two main ways to support our cells: nutrition and energy. Two ways that are available for everyone these days in almost any circumstance you may be in. I hope it will make you more conscious about the fact that there is more to our health than we are normally told by our regular doctors. That there are more ways to treat diseases and conditions than with drugs or surgery only. And that it is possible to help your body to use its selfhealing and -strengthening capabillities by focusing on supporting our cellular health.

In the last chapter of this book I will give you 25 more general tips for your health and nutrition that are based on good science and can easily be implemented in your daily life.

Chapter 1 : What is a cell?

We are in the age of having everything in the blink of an eye. We want it, and we want it now! We are fine with settling for the sausage biscuit for breakfast and the cheeseburger for lunch. We have done it consistently for so long that it is now routine, and our body has paid the price. Yes, our body has paid the price with its weakened cells, the building blocks of the body. But what exactly is a cell?

A cell is the smallest unit of life. Our body is made up of a large number of these cells, approximately 40 trillion cells. They are the basic structural, functional, and biological units our body is made up of.

A cell has a membrane on the outside and all the machinery to drive the metabolism on the inside. Cells provide the basic structure and function of all living things. For us humans, our cells are home to machines - DNA, RNA, proteins, lipids, mitochondria - that feed all complex processes in the body.

Not all cells are exactly the same, but almost all have the fundamental organization in common. Within the cell there is a nucleus, which has DNA. There is the cytoplasm where proteins are produced and there are mitochondria, which produce energy for the cell.

There are around 200 different types of human cells - blood cells, skin cells, nerve cells and more - responsible for different elements of your cellular health. For example, a brain cell uses electrochemical signals to process information, while a red blood cell carries oxygen to the tissues. In addition to their specialized functions, cell types also differ in the frequency of regeneration. Brain and heart cells, for example, regenerate slowly, if ever. The cells in your intestines spin every week.

A cell is composed of further small elements which include various organelles like the nucleus, Golgi apparatus, mitochondria, chloroplasts, peroxisomes and lysosomes, endoplasmic reticulum, centrosomes and vacuoles enveloped by a thin layer called cell membrane. Except for the nucleus and its contents, all others comprise the cytoplasm. All the biochemical processes take place in the cell when these organelles work together in collaboration as a function. Any disruption to any component of the cell can bring about disorientation which may lead to altered activity. This affects the health of the system to which the cell belongs. If a cell in your lungs for example disfunctions, a lung disease may be the result.

Now, you know the components of the cell I will tell you about the activities carried out by the most important organelles and how they work in association with eachother. This is the most difficult part of the book to understand, but it shows how complex but also intelligently our body works.

Body Cell

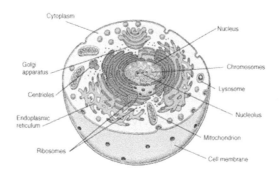

- Nucleus: It is the centre of the cell which stores all the information about the cell. It also contains the genetic information of the cell since it is the house of chromosomes where the DNA replication and RNA transcription takes place. An envelope called the nuclear envelope separates it from the cytoplasm. It contains the nucleolus which houses the subunits for RNA transcription. DNA replication involves the creation of its copy into a special RNA called the messenger RNA or simply mRNA. It is transported out of the nucleus, for its translation into a specific protein molecule.

- Mitochondria: This is the powerhouse of the cell. Here, the generation of the source of energy called ATP is generated by oxidative phosphorylation using oxygen. This ATP is the source of energy which is used up for all the biochemical reactions occurring in our bodies. They vary in number and are self-replicating.

- Endoplasmic reticulum (ER): They form the connecting links between molecules during processes of modification. The rough ER has ribosomes which secrete proteins into the ER. And the smooth ER lacks ribosomes and are mainly involved in the sequestration and the release of calcium.

- Golgi apparatus: The synthesis of proteins and lipids take place in the cells. Golgi apparatus processes and packs these molecules to be transported to their destinations.

- Lysosomes and Peroxisomes: These are the scavengers for worn out or excessive cell material. Lysosomes contain the enzymes called acid hydrolases which help the cell rid of the worn-out material by hydrolysing them and converting to excretory molecules. The enzymes stored in peroxisomes are the ones that help the cells get rid of free radicals such as peroxides.

- Centrosome: Its job is to organize. It provides directions for transportation to the Golgi apparatus and the ER.

- Vacuoles: They are several in number. Their job is to hold the excretory material until excreted.

DNA is housed in the cell's nucleus. It is different for every individual and genetic printing can be traced to identify the parents and children through DNA screening. So, if you have any traits matching your parents or grandparents or forefathers, then the information has passed from them to you through this genetic material, DNA.

The cell membrane around the cells is not the only lipid membrane in the body. In each of your cells, there is a smaller spherical nuclear membrane within which your DNA is stored. This way, your cell separates the DNA from the rest of the activities of your cell, such as the production of energy and the generation of proteins (synthesis), carried out in the cytoplasm.

DNA consists of nitrogen-based nucleotides connected to sugar and phosphate molecules. They are arranged in filaments in a helix formation, which develops to create a small intermediate molecule, called RNA, which carries DNA information throughth nuclear membrane to the cytoplasm where it can be read. From the instructions provided by the RNA, new proteins are synthesized. Specific areas of DNA that provide code for individual proteins are known as genes, and genes are organized into structures called chromosomes.

Your DNA never leaves the core, so the nuclear membrane is very important to declare your DNA. Unfortunately, your DNA can easily be damaged by a number of different factors. Toxins, especially fat soluble ones, like many pesticides, can pass through both cells and nuclear membranes. When they do, they can adhere to DNA, causing the loss of the shape or rupture of a filament. Damage can also occur from compounds called reactive oxygen species (ROS), a type of Free Radical, which are toxic by-products of damaged energy production. DNA damage of this type is called mutation. Mutations can lead to altering cell programming, sometimes turning a healthycell into a tumor cell.

It's vital to protect the shield of your DNA. When your strands break and your structure is compromised, not only are you not able to make the right types and amounts of proteins needed for the proper functioning of your body, but these mutations can lead to cancer. Supporting healthy membranes by eating foods that provide unsaturated inlet and avoiding those containing saturated and trans fatty acids is a way to declare DNA. Eating organic food is another way because it minimizes exposure to pesticide residues in food. Minimizing the use of pesticides not only in agriculture, but also in our lawngand flowerbeds, and supporting companies that do not use toxic compoundsfrom the environment is another way to declare DNA from damage. Finally adding the right frequencies and energy to your cells is a good way to help your DNA to stay healthy.

Keeping dietary levels of protein to be adeⵧuate and antioxidant vitamins such as vitamins E and C are also important for the health of your DNA, as well as to support the production of healthy energy by reducing the amount of damaging free radicals within the cells. Nutritional support for healthy DNA also includes adequate dietary intake of folate and vitamin B12, as these micronutrients are involved in DNA replication and repair. Folate is present in high concentrations of green leaf tea, cereals and eggs. And vitamin B12 can be obtained from eggs, dairy products, meat and fish.

Chapter 2 : Cellular Health

Our cells are now not as strong as you may think. They cannot fight the free radicals that we take in everyday. The body is under constant attack from oxidative stress. Oxygen in the body splits into single atoms with unpaired electrons. Electrons like to be in pairs, so these atoms, called free radicals, scavenge the body to seek out other electrons so they can become a pair. This causes damage to cells, proteins and DNA. The natural production of antioxidants is not enough to fight these free radicals. This is where cellular nutrition comes in. Cellular nutrition helps to fight free radicals that we are taking in every day at a phenomenal rate due to the increase of environmental pollution, poor diets, airborne toxins, medications, drinking and smoking, just to name a few. Cellular nutrition actually begins to start repairing the body at its cellular core.

The process begins in your small intestines. There live villi (tinyfinger-like protrusions). If you were to spread your fingers wide open and wiggle them, it would give you a general idea of healthy villi. This is where our bodies absorbs all the nutrients from food and vitamins that we intake.

When the villi become damaged, they begin to close up. Their function, becomes minimal and strained. Image those spread out wiggling fingers now closed up into a fist like position. This is the breakdown of your villi. Over the years, they will absorb less and less of the nutrients we need, our bodies will begin to breakdown, and we will feel worse and worse as time moves forward. Our bodies are also fooled into thinking that we are starving because the nutrients we are getting are not getting to the villi it needs to be healthy.

We begin to crave sugars and fats, as they are the easiest for our bodies to absorb. The fats and sugars then tend to make we feel more fatigued and tired. Our bodies then store the fat because it believes it is starving. If you are trying to lose weight, this will be almost impossible. Your body is in the mode of storing fat, not burning it.

Basically, the health of any cell and even any organism is dependent on the two factors. These are:

1. Nutrition

2. Energy

Nutrition that goes in will determine the functioning of any cell and the organism in turn. Proper nutrition is the basic core of nourishment. If nutrition is not good, proper functioning can never be carried out. With our current lifestyles, the nutrition part has been highly neglected. It is questionable how any cell suffering malnutrition can even derive the energy required for a person's body to stay in function. It is with the right nutrition only that the biochemical processes occurring in each cell are able to perform well. It is always the lack of right nutrition and energy at this basic cell level that hampers our health.

It is important to know how you can improve your cellular health in order to improve your overall health. What I can say simply is that we need to find the underlying root cause of any problem. Our unhealthy lifestyle and people around me suffering from serious diseases have made me conscious about my own health and made me write this guide. I want as many people as possible out there to live healthy lives. I want you to know how you can prevent various disease threats by changing your lifestyle and better nutrition. Apart from this, it is the lack of general knowledge about cellular health that makes you ignorant of the threats. So, you need to understand the basic functioning of our systems at the cellular level to be able to live a healthier life.

Improving Cellular Health

Our body is made up of billions of cells. Without them, vital organs will not work. In fact, their non-existence will probably wipe humankind off the surface of the earth. Needless to say, cells are essential for our health.

Ironically, we usually neglect the minute things. We normally only think about the health of our large organs. But we do not pay close attention to the health of our tiny cells. But actually this is where most of our diseases start.

When we are exposed to the sun's UV rays, smoke, pollution, stress and toxins, our body undergoes a chemical oxidation process. This oxidation process triggers the release of harmful free radicals. These are single electrons that roam freely in the body. They are called free radicals because they follow a free pathway. They are harmful because of they damage cells.

While roaming, they meet paired electrons along the way. When they get into contact with those paired electrons, they tend to snatch up an electron so they can have a pair. This leads to cellular and DNA damage. In the previous chapter we saw what this damage can lead to.

In the next chapters I will talk about cellular health in comparison to convential medicine (by our "regular" doctors), about cellular health and nutrition and cellular health and energy. That last subject is probably most unknown to people but offers amazing possibilities for the future.

Chapter 3 : Cellular Health in Comparison to Conventional Health

The cells are the cornerstones of their own existence. Being healthy and buzzing are key to preventing ageing and disease. But have you ever talked to your doctor about your cells?

We're used to thinking about our health, macro-level. We often take bloodpressure, temperature or weight into account when assessing our health. But scientists know that health is determined by the basic components of your body cells.

Cell health is important because it determines the health of each organ, which consists of cells. The cell is in a sense the unit of health of our organs and with that of our body. All ageing and disease begin at the cellular level, and often cell function deteriorates before you realize that something is out. This means that thinking about our health at the microlevel can make an important contribution to maintaining good health. Furthermore many diseases that start in the cells are not being felt in the body before it may be too late. Cancer is one of the most frightening examples of this.

Cellular health as defined above is a more natural way in keeping the overall health condition of the body in check. Our conventional system of medicine includes the use of drugs, surgery and radiations to treat the diseases and their symptoms by healthcare professionals. But these systems do not go anywhere near the depth of the underlying condition, which is the cellular level. So what is needed is to shift the approach of treatment by bringing about a shift in the paradigm. More and more research shows that our medicine dominated by big pharmaceutical companies is not sufficient to really face the health challenges the human race meets. We need that focus on the cells for prevention but also in some cases to treat diseases more effectively.

Many people have already been transforming in the way they look for alternative treatment options. They are driven by their values, beliefs, and philosophical orientations toward health and life. Recent results have revealed more people going into looking for alternative medicines. Alternative medicine that often is based on wisdom that has been around for hundreds and even thousands of years. More and more we recoqnize the value of for example Indian and Chinese medicine.

So why do people finally understand that it is their own responsiblillity to understand and control their health and not their doctor's?

- Dissatisfaction: People who have been on conventional treatments or have seen them close enough also know about their unwanted (side) effects, the high cost, the impersonal touch and sometimes the lack of results. While cellular health can be seen as a personalized treatment that can improve the health at the base functional level without causing any adverse effects and at the same time being affordable. Though conventional medicine systems seem to be an option in case of emergency treatments, they too can be transformed to cellular level or at least work in association to befit all medical situations.

- Personal control: People seek personal autonomy and control over their health care decisions. With an impersonal touch of conventional medicines, patients lose faith. They want some personalized treatment alternatives which lead them to come across other methods that can treat their underlying condition.

- Philosophical congruence: Alternative therapies seem an attraction for being more compatible with patients' values, spiritual/religious beliefs and myths regarding the nature of health and illness.

Our "western" medicine has gone through an amazing development in the last 50 years. Technology has helped us to understand diseases better and organize care and cure as efficiently and effectively as possible. Our healthcare professionals are well trained and motivated to help us. We can be thankful that we can profit from all of this. But that is not enough. In our modern society we are confronted with diseases that we did not know a hundred years ago. Partly because of the way we live but also because of the focus on the symptoms and not the causes. Therefor I plead for more insight into the working of our cells and our cellular health. Not tot replace conventional medicine but to enrich it.

Chapter 4 : Cellular Health and Nutrition

According to many studies cellular damage contributes to the appearance of numerous diseases such as Cancer and Alzheimer's disease. Moreover, it also makes our skin look older. Unhealthy cells speed up the appearance of wrinkles and fine lines. If you want to look younger, you should improve cellular health.

To illustrate more clearly how nutrition benefits cellular health, we see the function of three of its cellular components: (1) the cell membrane, (2) the nucleus and (3) the mitochondria, and we see how nutrition influences its structure, function and integrity. This will allow you to better understand how different nutrients in your diet can help promote the health of your cells, and thus the health of your entire being.

Why are healthy foods so good for my cells?

As can be seen from previous chapters, support for healthy cells involves a variety of vitamins and minerals, as well as other food components. Providing all these nutrients to cells means eating whole foods as they contain the most complete complement of these nutrients. One of the most complete sources of food for nutrients that support healthy cells is whole grains.

Because bread is such an important part of most of our diets I pay some extra attention to the importance of whole grains.

An entire grain, such as a grain of wheat contains three main parts: bran, germ and endosperm. The bran is the outer layer and is rich in fiber. The germ is the inner layer and is rich in nutrients. The endosperm is the bulk of the kernel and contains some of the vitamins and minerals. Whole grains contain all three parts of this kernel. Refining normally removes the bran and the germ, leaving only the endosperm. Without the bran and germ, about 25% of a grain's protein is lost, and are greatly reduced in at least seventeen key nutrients. Processors add back some vitamins and minerals to enrich refined grains, so refined products still contribute valuable nutrients. But whole grains are healthier, providing more protein, more fiber and many important vitamins and minerals.

Each part of the grain has different goals, and therefore a different nutritional supplement. The germ is rich in micronutrients. It contains a high level of vitamin E, tocopherols and several B vitamins.

The endosperm, although it is most of the grain, contains the least amount of micronutrients because of its size, as its purpose is simply to provide calories from starch (sugar). The bran contains over 60% of the minerals found in grains, including magnesium, the amino acid, the potassium, the iron, copper and manganese. All of which are necessary to maintain healthy cells. It is easy to understand why whole grains get so much attention in health publications, because the products of processed grains, like white bread and refined grains, provide only little protection against cell damage.

Your cells need a full range of vitamins, especially B vitamins, to support energy production and keep the level of free radicals to a minimum. Your cells also need omega-3 fatty acids and a good source of protein to support healthy and protective membranes. And your cells need a high intake of antioxidants such as the compounds of vitamin E found in the germs of whole grains, vitamin C found in citrus fruits, and carotenoids of plants to fight against the free radical damage to your DNA. A number of other nutrients can also act as antioxidants and help the prevention of damage to DNA by free radicals. These include fruit anthocyanidi, such as grapes and strawberries, and catechins found in green tea and fruits such as grapes.

Without this support of nutrients, cell membranes can become fragile, develop holes (torture), not be able to function properly, and not be protective for the DNA of their cells and energy production machines. Once unprotected, DNA can develop mutations that can make the cell unable to function, or even become cancerous. The damage to your machine and producer of energy can decrease the production of energy and lead to an increase in the generation of free radicals, causing more damage and destroying the ability of your cell to function fully.

The envelope that surrounds the cell is called the cell membrane. The cell membrane acts as a structural boundary that surrounds each of its cells and protects its internal mechanism (such as energy-producing reactions), so that they can function properly. It also serves as a filter, semi-permeable, through which nutrients can enter and waste can be eliminated, and allows cells to communicate with each other, allowing the orchestration of all physiological functions of your body.

The cell membrane is composed primarily of fat. It's like a drop of oil in the blood and tissue. Entering, being insoluble in water, forms a barrier that gives its cells their limits and structure. The main function of entering your cell membrane is to create structural shape and stability. Many of the entrants that make up the membrane are known as losumanolipids, which are a combination of fatty acids, a carbon structure to which they are linked called glyercol, and phosphate.

Proteins in cell membranes are important for many cell functions. Proteins are also an important component of cells. Outside cells, proteins make up bones and soft tissues and help these structures maintain their shape. Because they can be done in many different shapes and sizes, and they also make digestive enzymes, antibodies in the blood, and serve many other functions. Proteins have many functions within cells. They provide all the enzymatic functions for energy production; they repair DNA when it is damaged, and with input, they maintain the integrity of the cell membrane. Proteins are found in the cell membrane, in the cell itself, and around the cells.

The proteins that make up the cell membrane serve a variety of important purposes, such as communication between cells, and provide attack sites, so that cells can stone with surrounding structures and remain where they should. For example, bone cells bind to the bone matrix through proteins in their cell membranes, and liver cells remain in the liver by binding to liver tissue through specific binding proteins in their cell membranes. Cancer cells often have changes in these proteins attached to their membranes, which affect their ability to "stick" or stay where they should, allowing them to move around the body. Therefore, proteins in the cell membrane are important not only for the functioning of the individual cell, but also for the health of the whole body.

Your cells must communicate constantly with each other, absorbing nutrients from the bloodstream and wasting excrement. Cells do this by having proteins that respond to body signals nailed to each of their membranes. These proteins act as channels that can be opened or closed when your cell receives a signal to do so, or as carriers of information, as a telegraph line through its membrane, to communicate what is happening outside or inside the neighboring cells. This communication is vital to your ability to function as an entire body with all the cells working together.

For example, think about when you eat a meal. Sugar (glucose) is released and inserted into the body through the digestion process, during which it enters the blood. The body reacts to glucose in the blood by secreting insulin from the pancreas into the bloodstream. When insulin reaches one of its cells that needs glucose, it binds to a protein (receptor) on the cell surface, which then activates, or opens, a door in the cell to get glucose in that cell. This glucose is then used by the cell to produce energy or stored for the future of energy production.

Nutrients in the foods you eat can promote healthy cell membranes. Research has shown that nutrients absorbed through the diet can have a significant influence on the health of cell membranes. The incoming unsaturated fats, such as omega-3 fatty acids found in fish and nuts, are necessary for cell membranes to have their form and the ability to communicate. Research studies on the other hand show that trans and saturated fats in the cell membrane make the cells less able to communicate and respond to signals; it is as if the cell membranes become brittle.

Consuming healthy levels of unsaturated food, especially omega-3 fatty acids, and avoiding trans and saturated inlets is a way to support healthy cell membranes. Inositol and choline are two other food compounds that are also components of cell membranes and promote cell function. Inositol, which helps carry signals through cell membranes, is found in cereals, such as wheat or brown rice. Studies have shown an association between the highest levels of inositol ingestion and a lower risk of cancer, such as colon cancer, which may be due to the function of inositol in supporting healthy cell membranes.

Cereals, vegetables, and fruits also contain many molecules that help prevent cell membranes to be damaged. These nutrients are protective and include the family of molecules of vitamin E, called tocopherols, that are found in higher concentrations in oils of cereals, such as wheat germ oil; carotenoids such as beta-carotene in carrots and lycopene in tomatoes; vitamin C in citrus fruits.

One of the things many people overlook when thinking about theirs cells is cellular ageing. This is probably because it goes undetected. You can't really see the symptoms of cellular ageing.

When the body undergoes a chemical oxidation process, the fat reserves produce harmful free radicals. Free radicals are single electrons that follow a free pattern. When they meet paired electrons, they tend to snatch one to pair up with. This disturbs cellular and DNA functions.

The improper functions of cells can contribute to the appearance of several debilitating illnesses such as Cancer. The more obvious signs of cell ageing are seen on our skin. Your skin will look dull, flaky and lifeless.

One of the best ways to combat this form of ageing is through antioxidants. Antioxidants are molecules that prevent cellular oxidation. These molecules also repair the damages caused by harmful free radicals.

You can find antioxidants from natural sources such as fruits and vegetables. Citrus fruits such as kiwi, Asian pear, oranges and apples contain vitamins that also work as antioxidants. Berries like strawberries and blueberries also contain antioxidants.

You can also find antioxidants in supplement form. A supplement that has shown to reduce oxidative stress with at least 40% is Protandim. Protandim is a food supplement based on five natural products. The five ingredients are: Turmeric, Bacopa, Green Tea, Ashwagandha and Milk Thistle. Protandim is the only supplement proven in a clinical study to reduce oxidative stress by an average of 40% in 30 days. Protandim has been shown to increase superoxide dismutase levels by 30%, glutathione by 300%, and catalase by 54%. When individuals were supplemented with Protandim for 30 days, the age-dependent increase in lipid peroxidation was completely eliminated. Lipid peroxidation in an older person was reduced to the level of a 20-year-old. This means the body is not only capable of making its own antioxidant enzymes, but also that their production can be activated by Protandim to reduce cellular stress and may help protect against the aging process and several conditions in which cellular stress has been reported to be a contributing factor.

Energy supply and production: mitochondria

The cell membrane surrounds the cells, like the skin around your body. Like your body has tissues and organs to support your general function, each of your cells has its own miniature version of the tissues and organs. Miniaturized organs are called organelles, and perform most of the daily functions in their cell. Some of the most important organelles in your cells are energy plants, called mitochondria.

Mitochondria are where cells produce the energy they need from the nutrients in the food they eat. Each of your cells has several hundred up to more than two thousand mitochondria within them, depending on your energy needs. For example, heart cells and skeletal muscle cells, which have a high energy requirement to support constant movements in the body, have up to 40% of their space occupied by mitochondria. In total, your body has more than a quadrillion mitochondria that constantly produce energy.

Mitochondria use oxygen and nutrients from the food they eat to produce energy. Most of the energy produced by your mitochondria comes from the degradation of glucose or fat in your diet. Since mitochondria produce the energy used by other parts of the cells and throughout the body, they must have a way to transport that energy. They do this using a molecule called adenosine triphosphate, or ATP. ATP can be produced in one part of the cell and transported to another place where the energy has" passed".

The ATP carries energy through a high-energy phosphate that is removed from the site where its energy is used. When ATP abandons, or "expands" its energy, as when muscles need energy to move, this high-energy phosphate is removed from ATP, and becomes adenosine diphosphate, or ADP. The ADP is then brought back to its mitochondria, where it can have another high-energy phosphate put in it to form the ATP again, and so-as an energy shuttle that moves the energy forward and backward is used and reused for energy transport.

On an average day, when you do nothing in particular, you will use the equivalent of about half of what you weigh on ATP. About 90% of the oxygen you breathe is used by your mitochondria to produce this energy. As ATP is recycled ADP and then converted to ATP to transport more energy, it will not gain or lose weight in this energy production process. Energy production uses a multitude of nutrients, as well as many other food molecules. Let's take a closer look at the chemical reactions involved in energy production and the role of these nutrients in ATP production.

The attachment of high-energy phosphate to ADP to form ATP is a complex process, as energy is the basis of everything that is happening in your body and it is what drives life to its most basic level. Mitochondria are like cells inside cells; they have their own membrane like the membrane of the cell. However each mitochondria has two membranes, one internal and one external. Its internal membrane is up to 75% protein, much more than any other membrane in its cell. These proteins are part of the electron transport chain (ETC) and play a key role in the production of ATP.

The food you eat must first be prepared for the ETC. For this, the body takes glucose or the fat molecule and breaks it down into smaller units. These two-carbon units are then stripped of some units of energy, called electrons, and decomposed into carbon dioxide, which is transported out of mitochondria as waste. A small amount of energy is generated during this process, which is called the Kreb cycle. The main role of the Kreb cycle, however, is to break electrons from glucose and enter into energy production by the ETC, which will generate the greatest amount of energy. The cycle of

Kreb uses a multitude of vitamins and minerals, especially vitamins B1, B2, B3, B5 and B6; and this is one of the reasons the B vitamins are considered vitamins for energy.

The mitochondria use molecules made of B2 and B3 vitamins to transfer electrons from the Kreb cycle to ETC, because the remaining unprotected electrons damage the components of their cell. It moves, or transmits these electrons through a chain of proteins, almost like a river of electrons where proteins are the banks of the river. Electrons settle at the end of the protein chain within the double membrane in the mitochondria, creating an electron gradient, like a reservoir of dams at the end of a river. ETC uses five enzyme complexes in its membrane to create this electron tank, and also burns oxygen as part of this process. At the end of ETC is the energy barrier, or the door that, when opened, allows electrons to pass through and, like a barrier, transfers energy to create ATP. In the center of the ETC is the nutrient coenzyme Q10, which is very important for electron transport and membrane protection. The ETC is made up of proteins that require iron and sulfur, nutrients that are also needed to get from the foods you eat. Iron is present in whole grains, and good sources of sulfur are cruciferous vegetables, such as broccoli.

Maintaining the structural integrity of your mitochondria is fundamentally important for your overall health and well-being. If tissues and organs, especially those that most need energy, such as muscles, heart, and brain, do not receive enough energy, they cannot function properly. Therefore, mitochondrial dysfunction is considered one of the main basic factors of unhealthy aging and fatigue. Mitochondrial dysfunction is also an important factor in many chronic degenerative diseases, such as congestive heart failure and diabetes. In addition to the inability to produce energy, if damaged, mitochondria can also produce harmful by-products, such as reactive oxygen species, a type of radical species that can destroy DNA and proteins.

Nutritional support for healthy energy production includes support for healthy membranes. In addition, because B vitamins are so important, sufficient intake of B1, B2, B3, B5 and B6 vitamins is extremely important to support energy metabolism. Good sources of these vitamins include whole grains, as B vitamins are concentrated in cereal Bran. Whole grains are an excellent source of all B vitamins related to energy. Wheat germ is one of the highest sources of tocopherols, the vitamin family and micronutrients, and brown rice contains orizanol and ferulic acid, known as

effective antioxidants and health-promoting
compounds.

Chapter 5 : Electromedicine, Energy and Frequencies

In the previous chapter I described the importance of energy for the body. Our body has the possibillitiy to produce its own energy through the mitochondria resulting in ATP. This ATP is vital for the need of energy our has body has. Unfortunately there are many reasons why our body is not able to produce enough energy. The main reason is that our cells do not get enough or the right nutrients. But there is also a way to directly "upload" energy into your cells. This way is called electromedicine.

Electromedicine is defined as a discipline within the field of medicine that uses electronics and energy technologies to aid in the treatment of a variety of physical symptoms, ailments and disease conditions.

Electromedicine recognizes that the body is primarily electric and some form of electricity is found naturally in all of us and controls the function of every cell of our bodies and that a wide variety of electrical impulses in our bodies help facilitate all bodily functions including all actions needed for health maintenance, healing and regeneration.

By transmitting and conditioning the cells of the body with harmonic electrical impulses that occur in a perfect state of energetic health, we can help balance and direct these impulses.

Although electromedicine has been around since the late 1800's, the control and profits of conventional medicine, namely surgery and drugs, has overshadowed and forced into the background many viable alternatives and treatments that offer, many times, better results and, most times, less side effects.

The historic advances in electromedicine technology make it a safer, and more noticeably effective alternative. Some of the latest technologies have enabled us to see noticeable improvement in a wider variety of symptoms and in more serious conditions. The most advanced, like the TimeWaver and Healy, have become a significant complement to other therapies without negative side effects.

In this chapter I will take you through the history of electromedicine and I will touch topics like biochemistry, biophysics, bioresonance, frequency specific microcurrent and information field.

Electromedicine – Early years

Electromedicine was first documented in 1890 at the American Electro-Therapeutic Association's annual conferences on the therapeutic use of electricity and electrical devices by physicians on ailing patients.

Since 1890, electromedicine has evolved significantly:

- Nikola Tesla - in 1895 discovered alternating current and invented the AC generator, published many papers, and invented numerous electrical devices including Tesla coil therapy instruments.

- Alexander Gurvich - in 1922 discovered "biophotons" and "mitogenic" "mitotic" waves. His work is the first documented evidence of "biophotons," and became the basis for the design of later bioelectromagnetic therapy devices.

- Georges Lakhovsky - in 1925 invented the multi-wave oscillator which produced a spectrum of electrical frequencies that restored cell equilibrium in the body, and published a paper in "Radio News" magazine titled "Curing Cancer with Ultra Radio Fre□uencies."

- Royal Raymond Rife - in the 1930's demonstrated how his frequency research and mitogenic impulse-wave technology (specifications in public domain) could cure cancer.

- Ed Skilling - 1950's break through discoveries with space-age electronics, transmission and communication with the cells and the body's immune system; results supercede all prior electromedicine technologies.

Quantum Leap in Electromedicine

Ed Skilling's work with advanced electronics in the late 1950's leads to a ⬚uantum leap in electromedicine. His discoveries take the results of electromedicine to a new and profound level by communicating with the cells of the body using harmonic energy impulses and by introducing the harmonic balance and flow of life-force energy throughout the body.

Prior electromedicine technology including Rife specifications (still used today) works with "frequencies" that do not penetrate the body at the cellular level. The difficulty is in the way our bodies are created.

The human body is created "resistant" to protect us from things flying around the universe such as ultra-violet rays and microwaves, etc. The proof is in the way we can lay out in 100 plus degree sun and burn our skin and not hurt our brain, liver, kidneys, or internal organs.

While this is a blessing that protects us all, it is a problem in treating, reaching and improving internal organs and functions of the body. This is primarily why past technologies that basically "zapped" the surface of the body got limited results that were not consistent for everyone.

Skilling's breakthrough technology changes this and improves results more noticeably than any technologies of the past. His technology transmits life-force energy (the kind of energy in the cells, and natural cellular energy that the cells use to communicate with each other) and achieves energetic communication with all the organs and systems of the body at the cellular level in harmony with the "impedance" (resistance) of the body.

Integrating Biochemistry and Biophysics

Since the 1950's more and more research was done and new insights into electromedicine followed quickly. Three important researchers were:

- Robert O. Becker, MD, an orthopedist/researcher at the State University of New York, spent more than 30 years attempting to determine how trillions of cells, with hundreds of subtypes, can function harmoniously in life. He found that a primitive direct current data transmission and control system exists in biological systems for the regulation of growth and healing. He calls this the fourth nervous system. Becker has laid the groundwork for the medical professions to start to evolve towards a more reasonable integrated view of biology, incorporating our understanding of both biochemistry and biophysics.

- Björn Nordenström, MD, Emeritus Professor of Radiology at Karolinska Institute in Stockholm who also served as Chairman of the Nobel Assembly, has proposed a new and distinct model of bioelectrical control systems he calls biologically closed electric circuits (BCEC). Nordenström's theory is that the mechanical blood circulation system is closely integrated anatomically and physiologically with a bioelectrical system. The principle is similar to closed circuits in electronic technology.

- Ngok Chang, MD, of the Department of Biochemistry and Orthopedic Surgery at the University of Louvain, Belgium proposed another mechanism. His research showed that microcurrent stimulation increased adenosine triphosphate (ATP) generation by almost 500 percent. Increasing the level of current to milliampere levels actually decreased the results. Microcurrent was also shown to enhance amino acid transport and protein synthesis in the treated area 30 to 40 percent above controls.

The cytologists Dr. Robert O. Becker and Dr. Bjorn Nordenstrom, former chairman of the Nobel Prize Committee, found out that almost all acute and chronic diseases may be caused by a decrease in the cell's membrane voltage.

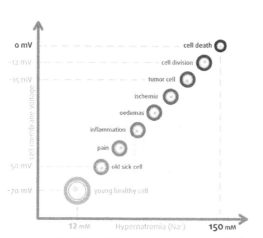

In case of a decreased cell membrane voltage, the number of sodium ions (Na⁺) increases in the cell. This phenomenon is called hypernatremia.

According to their model, a person is just as healthy as his or her cells and their ability to communicate with each other. Thus, the health of the cell can be linked to this simple parameter: the electric cell membrane voltage. If ideally, the cell has a voltage of -70 mV, it has enough energy to live and to communicate with other cells. In the course of disease processes this voltage often decreases to -50 mV. In case of a voltage of -40 mV, pain and inflammation may arise. According to Becker and

Nordenstrom, -15 mV is the threshold where the cell can mutate to a tumor cell.

Transcutaneous electrical nerve stimulation (TENS) came on the scene in the 1970s following Melzack and Wall's introduction of the Gate Control Theory of pain in 1965 in which counter stimulation could effectively close the gate to peripheral pain messages attempting to ascend spinal pathways to the brain. TENS stimulation is typically applied at a level of 60 or more milliamperes of current. Nearly 50 years later, microcurrent electrical therapy now aims at altering or eliminating the pain message by normalization of the cell function. With bioresonance a next step was taken towards a wider use of electromedicine to care and even (in some cases) cure.

Bioresonance therapy is a treatment which can be used to diagnose and cure a range of illnesses. Also known as electrodermal testing, bio-energetic therapy, and vibrational medicine, bioresonance operates on the same principle as energetic healing. It is non-invasive, natural and boasts astounding results.

The science of bioresonance treats illnesses using electromagnetic frequencies. These frequencies harmonize the bioresonance of your body and its organs. Once restored, a rapid process of self-healing is started. Restoring your resonance restores your internal balance allowing all your organs to function as they should.

This form of treatment began life as a therapy developed by Franz Morell and Erich Rasche. Initially termed MORA therapy (MORell & RAsche), this treatment began life in Germany in the 1970s. The first MORA-Therapy instrument was developed as an all-embracing holistic technology based on sound scientific foundational theory. It holds roots in acupuncture and homeopathy as well as anatomy and pathology. Dr. Franz Morell determined that each organ has a specific oscillation spectrum. This oscillation spectrum is detectable and measurable as a resonant magnetic frequency. The body encompasses many natural harmonic frequencies. Each one can be isolated individually and as part of a larger system.

We are all vibrational beings sharing a magnetic resonance at a quantum level. Even planet earth emits a measurable frequency termed the Schumann Resonance. Our environment and lifestyle effects the vibrational frequency emitted. A bioresonance machine can be used to scan the body. This can identify everything from biological imbalances to objects, food types and other environmental allergens which disturb your biological harmony. It is this harmony which is fundamental for our total well-being. Bioresonance therapy corrects any interference patterns. Once corrected, your body reverts to its optimal state of self-rejuvenation.

A bioresonance therapy diagnostic procedure involves a reading from one of your meridians using a device which emits a magnetic circuit. Various electronic devices are used operating on similar principles as electroencephalography (EEG) and ultrasound. The intensity of your reading reveals key information concerning your health and body. Many of the imbalances which cause our disorders are connected ways which you would never expect.

An analysis of your bioresonance will reveal underlying connections at the root of poor health. Bioresonance therapy is an astonishingly effective treatment once discordant frequencies have been isolated. Electromagnetic impulses at precise ranges are sent to match and harmonize discordance, which stimulates the body to heal itself at a rapid rate thanks to the natural state it returns.

Bioresonance is being used and studied in various areas. Here are a few examples.

Smoking cessation

A 2014 study compared bioresonance used for smoking cessation to a placebo. It found that 77.2 percent of people in the bioresonance group quit smoking after one week after therapy versus 54.8 percent in the placebo group. The study also found that after a year from treatment — which was only done once — 28.6 percent of people in the bioresonance group had stopped smoking, versus 16.1 percent in the placebo group.

Stomach pain

Bioresonance has been used to treat stomach pain. One study found that this therapy was useful specifically for reducing stomach pain not associated with a specific diagnosis.

Allergies and related conditions

Using bioresonance to treat allergies and related conditions such as eczema and asthma is one of the most well-studied areas of bioresonance treatment. There have been a number of both controlled (using a placebo) and uncontrolled (observational) studies in this area. Controlled studies are generally considered of a higher caliber than uncontrolled studies due to their ability to compare treatment to a placebo.

Rheumatoid arthritis

Some studies suggest that bioresonance might be effective in rheumatoid arthritis (RA) by normalizing how antioxidants function within the body. These antioxidants help fight free radicals, which may help lessen tissue damage in people with RA. No formalized studies on the effectiveness of bioresonance in treating RA have been undertaken.

Fibromyalgia

One study compared the combination of bioresonance therapy, manual therapy, and point massage for treatment of fibromyalgia to manual therapy and point therapy without bioresonance therapy. While both groups saw improvement, the study found a 72 percent improvement in muscular pain for the group that got bioresonance therapy versus a 37 percent improvement for the other group. Improvements in sleep issues and sensitivity to weather changes were also found.

Frequency-specific microcurrent (FSM)

Caroline McMakin is the clinical director of the Fibromyalgia and Myofascial Pain Clinic of Portland, Oregon. She developed Frequency Specific Microcurrent

(FSM) in 1995. She used FSM to induce changes in inflammatory cytokines and substance P in the treatment of fibromyalgia associated with spine trauma, treatment of pain in the head, neck and face, and low back caused by myofascial trigger points, delayed onset muscle soreness, shingles and neuropathic pain.

FSM is a method employed for treating pain by using low-level electrical current delivered to certain parts of the body. A frequency is a rate at which a sound wave or electronic pulse is produced. It has been well researched that various frequencies can be used to potentially reduce inflammation (swelling), repair tissue, and reduce pain.

This method of frequency therapy focuses on the cellular level and is meant to lead to lasting success on the causal level. The human body produces its current within each cell. In FSM, depending on the tissue involved, specific frequencies are selected to encourage natural healing of the body and to reduce pain.

Chapter 6 : The Future of Cellular Health

The good health of the cells means that the importance of the molecules that make up cells, proteins, mitochondria and the DNA they work well and are free of damage, as long as the cells to function properly.

At a certain level, all diseases are dysfunctions that occur within cells. For example, when you have a cold, a virus infects the cells, causing symptoms such as low fever and nasal discharge. When you have Type 2 diabetes, your cells are no longer sensitive to insulin, resulting in an inability to drive your blood sugar.

But apart from diseases, what most affects cell health is time. Aging leads to a deterioration in cellular health. It seems ☐uite simple (of course, your cells degrade over time, right?), but it took hundreds of years of research- starting in 1665, when cells were first identified - for scientists to understand exactly what happens when they age.

But what happens with aging is that over time, the damage begins to exceed the capacity of the processes of repair to repair things, leading to a progressive accumulation of damage. In fact, aging is not just a process; it is a cascade of various changes that occur at the same time. A review published in 2013 in Cell magazine identified nine different characteristics of aging, such as "mitochondrial dysfunction" — that is, when the cell metabolic engine stops functioning correctly - and "cellular senescence" — when cells stop dividing as part of the biological process.

Each cell in your body is like the operating system of a phone, with many different parts that can (and do) decompose over time, which requires repair. One of the daily tasks of your cells, in addition to performing their specialized functions, is to repair themselves to ensure the proper functioning of the operating system.

We know that not smoking or protecting yourself from UV rays can help protect cells from damage. And we know that simple lifestyle changes, such as proper nutrition, regular exercise, and stress management, can pay off at the cellular level. But scientists are also beginning to understand how we can slow down, or perhaps even reverse, aging. For example, an interesting area of research focuses on sirtuins, a group of proteins responsible for cell stability, in the form of things like DNA expression. Called "Longevity genes", sirtuins, discovered only in the 1990s, are crucial to maintaining cellular health, but we know that they can only work with a coenzyme called nicotinamide adenine dinucleotide (NAD+). Scientists also know that NAD+ decreases over time, suggesting that pleading with NAD+ precursors might be a way to keep your sirtuins better and longer and thus keep your cells healthy even longer. LifeVantage, the company that makes the supplement Protandim, recently also introduced a NAD+ supplement. The three Protandim supplements now support your mitochondria, Nrf2 and NDA+.

What are the next steps in cell health research?

After many years of research, scientists have learned a lot about cell health and how we could maintain it, but there is still much to discover. In addition to things like nad+ supplements, scientists are trying to figure out how calorie restriction could play a role in slowing aging. A low-calorie diet increases sirtuini's activity. Part of this may be due to the fact that we have evolved to endure periods when food is scarce. And one way to do that is to make the animal more stress-resistant."

Another area that scientists are examining is how to treat cellular senescence with so-called senolytic therapies. Senescent cells are essentially cells that stand in the way. Scientists believe that if you can eliminate them, you will make the entire person healthier. And now there's an entire field based on trying to design drugs that can eliminate senescent cells. A 2018 study published in Nature Medicine, for example, found that a combination of two senolytic drugs prevented cell damage, delaying physical dysfunction and extending the useful life of adult mice.

Western universities are still teaching that life is based on a chemical model. Given the explosive growth in electrical technologies and our ever increasing understanding of physics, it is more realistic in this age to view biological processes on an electrochemical basis rather than on a chemical basis alone. Modern thinking on the subject far transcends the use of force in electromedical interventions. Scientific electromedicine has only evolved recently, over the past 50 years. This is due, in part, to advances in electrical technology and our understanding of biophysics as a distinct discipline from biochemistry.

Therefor I really believe that the future of cellular health lies in the further development of technology to support our cells to be as healthy and strong as possible to take care of the selfhealing powers our body has.

The main advantages of electromedicine are:

- Very low incidence of adverse effects.
- Relatively easy to learn.
- Can be administered by paramedical personnel or by

patients themselves at home.

- Expands the practitioner's clinical capability.
- Enhances the total efficacy of clinical efforts.
- A proven effective alternative therapy in cases refractive to conventional methods.
- Eliminates, or reduces, the need for addictive medications in chronic pain and stress syndromes and allows the limited use of necessary drugs where polypharmacy effects are not well tolerated.
- May be applied on a scheduled basis or as needed.
- Some technologies produce cumulative and long-term effects as healing ensues.
- Highly cost effective. Electromedical products are durable, and may be used for years.

Science has found much information on how the brain and nervous system work. Most of this research involves the action potential as the sole mechanism of the nerve impulse. This is a very sophisticated and complex system for the transfer of information throughout our body. It is helpful to compare this concept of the nervous system to a computer. The fundamental signal in both the computer and the nervous system is a digital one. Both systems transfer information represented by the number of pulses per unit of time. Information is also coded according to where the pulses originate, where they go and whether or not there is more than one channel of pulses feeding into an area. All our senses are based on this type of pulse system. Like a computer, the nervous system operates remarkably fast and can transfer large amounts of information as digital on and off data. Without signals or information going from the brain to those parts of the body where it is needed our body would not function. Even though your hand constantly has the capability to grasp something, it will only do that when your brain tells it to do so.

Someone who developed a vision on exploring the interaction between matter and consciousness, your cells and the information it needs, is Marcus Schmieke. Marcus Schmieke is the inventor and developer of the TimeWaver systems and was born in 1966 in Oldenburg, Germany.

His encounter with the physicist Burkhard Heim, as well as his work on his own books about science and consciousness – The Last Secret and the Field of Life – laid the theoretical foundation for the development of Information Field technology. Through an intensive examination of Heim's model of the 12 dimensional structure of the universe, Marcus Schmieke gained a deep understanding of the physical Information Field. Only energy does not make a material body, it needs information where the energy needs to interact. So, information level needs to be considered, what Schmieke calls the "Information field". Every body, every person according to Schmieke has an "Information field" and each quantum system has a specific resonance frequency and if you find the right frequencies, you can change the energetic and material state.

In 2007, on the basis of the work of Burkhard Heim, the Russian physicist Nikolai Kozyrev and other scientists, Marcus Schmieke developed the first TimeWaver system and thus brought Information Field technology into practical application for the first time. Within a very short period of time it proved to be a success in complementary medicine, and now TimeWaver systems are being increasingly used in areas such as business, family and personality development.

At the beginning of the 20th century already great physicists like Max Planck, Albert Einstein, Nils Bohr, Werner Heisenberg, Wolfgang Pauli have developed the theory of quantum physics, but the application of it in medicine has not been used much since. With the technical development of the TimeWaver including the the development of the treatment protocols and medical protocols, TimeWaver is applying quantum physics to the human body and to the human being as a whole and making it practical for making people healthy.

TimeWaver was developed until 2006 and it was pure quantum information technology, and the frequency technology we developed until 2011. At the end of 2011, Schmieke's first Frequency Therapy Device was published. He developed it together with the Portuguese researcher, doctor and owner of many clinics, Nuno Nina. He is still working with him to connect the TimeWaver technology to practinal clinical experience. TimeWaver combines powerful technology with the best clinical experience.

The company that has developed TimeWaver now also made a wearable medical device for home use called Healy. Healy is a Class IIa certified medical device for the treatment of chronic pain, fibromyalgia, skeletal pain and migraine as well as for the adjuvant therapy of mental illness such as depression, anxiety and associated sleep disorders. Healy uses individually determined frequencies to stimulate specific areas of the body. Healy contains frequency programs that help promote your health, vitality and overall wellbeing. Healy is meant help you to increase your vitality to improve the flow of your energy reserves and to activate your energy reservoirs.

Healy is compact and uses your smartphone to do a part of the work. All you need is to install the Healy App on your smartphone before using Healy. After you have installed the app, it will tell you exactly what to do next. You can see on your screen what programs are available. Once you have selected a specific program on the screen, you will see its total running time and you will be instructed which electrodes to apply. You can adjust the intensity of the program yourself while it is running.

A healthy body and mind means quality of life. That's why Healy offers a wide range of applications to help you stay fit, to bioenergetically regenerate and to reduce pain. Healy has individual programs grouped in program groups like: Pain / Psyche, Sleep, Mental Balance, Skin, Fitness, Meridians, Chakras, Bioenergetic Balance and Protection Programs.

With the Healy electromedicine has now reached the consumer. Slowly the focus of medicine will turn from medical professionals who decide about the health of people to people who take control over their own health and involve professionals for advice when needed. By paying attention to our cellular health we focus on the cause and not on the symptoms. It gives us the power to control our health at basic level: the cell.

Chapter 7 : 25 Things to Know About (Cellular) Health

It's easy to get confused when it comes to health, nutrition and lifestyle. With this book about cellular health it doesn't become easier. Even qualified experts often seem to hold opposing opinions when it comes to health and new or alternative approaches. To help you to start improving your health anyway here are 25 health and nutrition tips that are actually based on good science and can easily be implemented in your daily life.

1. Don't drink sugar calories

Sugary drinks are among the most fattening items you can put into your body. This is because your brain doesn't measure calories from liquid sugar the same way it does for solid food. Therefore, when you drink soda, you end up eating more total calories. Sugary drinks are strongly associated with obesity, type 2 diabetes, heart disease, and many other health problems). Keep in mind that certain fruit juices may be almost as bad as soda in this regard, as they sometimes contain just as much sugar. Their small amounts of antioxidants do not negate the sugar's harmful effects.

2. Eat nuts

Despite being high in fat, nuts are incredibly nutritious and healthy. They're loaded with magnesium, vitamin E, fiber, and various other nutrients. Studies demonstrate that nuts can help you lose weight and may help fight type 2 diabetes and heart disease. Additionally, your body doesn't absorb 10–15% of the calories in nuts. Some evidence also suggests that this food can boost metabolism. In one study, almonds were shown to increase weight loss by 62%, compared with complex carbs..

3. Avoid processed junk food (eat real food instead)

Processed junk food is incredibly unhealthy. These foods have been engineered to trigger your pleasure centers, so they trick your brain into overeating — even promoting food addiction in some people. They're usually low in fiber, protein, and micronutrients but high in unhealthy ingredients like added sugar and refined grains. Thus, they provide mostly empty calories.

4. Don't fear coffee

Coffee is very healthy. It's high in antioxidants, and studies have linked coffee intake to longevity and a reduced risk of type 2 diabetes, Parkinson's and Alzheimer's diseases, and numerous other illnesses.

5. Eat fatty fish

Fish is a great source of high-quality protein and healthy fat. This is particularly true of fatty fish, such as salmon, which is loaded with omega-3 fatty acids and various other nutrients. Studies show that people who eat the most fish have a lower risk of several conditions, including heart disease, dementia, and depression.

6. Get enough sleep

The importance of getting enough quality sleep cannot be overstated. Poor sleep can drive insulin resistance, disrupt your appetite hormones, and reduce your physical and mental performance. What's more, poor sleep is one of the strongest individual risk factors for weight gain and obesity. One study linked insufficient sleep to an 89% and 55% increased risk of obesity in children and adults, respectively.

7. Take care of your gut health with probiotics and fiber

The bacteria in your gut, collectively called the gut microbiota, are incredibly important for overall health. A disruption in gut bacteria is linked to some of the world's most serious chronic diseases, including obesity.

Good ways to improve gut health include eating probiotic foods like yogurt and sauerkraut, taking probiotic supplements, and eating plenty of fiber. Notably, fiber functions as fuel for your gut bacteria.

8. Drink some water, especially before meals

Drinking enough water can have numerous benefits. Surprisingly, it can boost the number of calories you burn. Two studies note that it can increase metabolism by 24–30% over 1–1.5 hours. This can amount to 96 additional calories burned if you drink 8.4 cups (2 liters) of water per day. The optimal time to drink it is before meals. One study showed that downing 2.1 cups (500 ml) of water 30 minutes before each meal increased weight loss by 44%.

9. Don't overcook or burn your meat

Meat can be a nutritious and healthy part of your diet. It's very high in protein and contains various important nutrients. However, problems occur when meat is overcooked or burnt. This can lead to the formation of harmful compounds that raise your risk of cancer. When you cook meat, make sure not to overcook or burn it.

10. Avoid bright lights before sleep

When you're exposed to bright lights in the evening, it may disrupt your production of the sleep hormone melatonin. One strategy is to use a pair of amber-tinted glasses that block blue light from entering your eyes in the evening. This allows melatonin to be produced as if it were completely dark, helping you sleep better.

11. Take vitamin D3 if you don't get much sun exposure

Sunlight is a great source of vitamin D. Yet, most people don't get enough sun exposure. In fact, about 41.6% of the U.S. population is deficient in this critical vitamin. If you're unable to get adequate sun exposure, vitamin D supplements are a good alternative. Their benefits include improved bone health, increased strength, reduced symptoms of depression, and a lower risk of cancer. Vitamin D may also help you live longer.

12. Eat vegetables and fruits

Vegetables and fruits are loaded with prebiotic fiber, vitamins, minerals, and many antioxidants, some of which have potent biological effects. Studies show that people who eat the most vegetables and fruits live longer and have a lower risk of heart disease, type 2 diabetes, obesity, and other illnesses.

13. Make sure to eat enough protein

Eating enough protein is vital for optimal health. What's more, this nutrient is particularly important for weight loss. High protein intake can boost metabolism significantly while making you feel full enough to automatically eat fewer calories. It can also reduce cravings and your desire to snack late at night. Sufficient protein intake has also been shown to lower blood sugar and blood pressure levels.

14. Do some cardio

Doing aerobic exercise, also called cardio, is one of the best things you can do for your mental and physical health. It's particularly effective at reducing belly fat, the harmful type of fat that builds up around your organs. Reduced belly fat should lead to major improvements in metabolic health.

15. Don't smoke or do drugs, and only drink in moderation

If you smoke or abuse drugs, tackle those problems first. Diet and exercise can wait. If you drink alcohol, do so in moderation and consider avoiding it completely if you tend to drink too much.

16. Use extra virgin olive oil

Extra virgin olive oil is one of the healthiest vegetable oils. It's loaded with heart-healthy monounsaturated fats and powerful antioxidants that can fight inflammation. Extra virgin olive oil benefits heart health, as people who consume it have a much lower risk of dying from heart attacks and strokes.

17. Don't eat a lot of refined carbs

Not all carbs are created equal. Refined carbs have been highly processed to remove their fiber. They're relatively low in nutrients and can harm your health when eaten in excess. Studies show that refined carbs are linked to overeating and numerous metabolic diseases.

18. Don't fear saturated fat

Saturated fat has been controversial. While it's true that saturated fat raises cholesterol levels, it also raises HDL (good) cholesterol and shrinks your LDL (bad) particles, which is linked to a lower risk of heart disease. New studies in hundreds of thousands of people have questioned the association between saturated fat intake and heart disease.

19. Lift heavy things

Lifting weights is one of the best things you can do to strengthen your muscles and improve your body composition. It also leads to massive improvements in metabolic health, including improved insulin sensitivity. The best approach is to lift weights, but doing bodyweight exercises can be just as effective.

20. Avoid artificial trans fats

Artificial trans fats are harmful, man-made fats that are strongly linked to inflammation and heart disease. While trans fats have been largely banned in the United States and elsewhere, the U.S. ban hasn't gone fully into effect — and some foods still contain them.

21. Use plenty of herbs and spices

Many incredibly healthy herbs and spices exist. For example, ginger and turmeric both have potent anti-inflammatory and antioxidant effects, leading to various health benefits. Due to their powerful benefits, you should try to include as many herbs and spices as possible in your diet.

22. Take care of your relationships

Social relationships are incredibly important not only for your mental well-being but also your physical health. Studies show that people who have close friends and family are healthier and live much longer than those who do not.

23. Track your food intake every now and then

The only way to know exactly how many calories you eat is to weigh your food and use a nutrition tracker. It's also essential to make sure that you're getting enough protein, fiber, and micronutrients. Studies reveal that people who track their food intake tend to be more successful at losing weight and sticking to a healthy diet.

24. If you have excess belly fat, get rid of it

Belly fat is particularly harmful. It accumulates around your organs and is strongly linked to metabolic disease. For this reason, your waist size may be a much stronger marker of your health than your weight. Cutting carbs and eating more protein and fiber are all excellent ways to get rid of belly fat.

25. Eat eggs, yolk and all

Whole eggs are so nutritious that they're often termed "nature's multivitamin."It's a myth that eggs are bad for you because of their cholesterol content. Studies show that they have no effect on blood cholesterol in the majority of people. Additionally, a massive review in 263,938 people found that egg intake had no association with heart disease risk.Instead, eggs are one of the planet's most nutritious foods. Notably, the yolk contains almost all of the healthy compounds.

The bottom line

A few simple steps can go a long way toward improving your lifestyle. Still, if you're trying to live a healthier life, don't just focus on the foods you eat. Exercise, sleep, and social relationships are also important and have a closer look at the importance of your cellular health.

Conclusion

In an ideal world, cellular health would automatically allow each of our cells to function, reproduce, and communicate properly. Cells would have ample nourishment and protection and be capable of completing the thousands of processes necessary for total and complete health.

Unfortunately, we live in a toxic world and the natural mechanisms designed to ensure cell health have been damaged. High-stress lifestyles, processed foods, chemicals in cleaning and personal care products, and excessive use of prescription drugs bombard our cells and make it difficult for these tiny—yet essential parts of our total health to perform properly.

We have different types of cells for each body system from nervous system function to elimination of toxins and bi-products. Each cell is dependent upon other cells in other systems to do its job, communicate, and collaborate. We don't feel these processes and often don't realize our cells are not working properly until major illness or disease sets in. Unfortunately, many of the life-stages we consider as a normal part of aging are in fact signs of cell degeneration and distress.

The good news is that modern science and nutrition understandings reveal that diet changes, supplementation, efforts to reduce toxicity and the use of modern electromedicine technology can increase overall health, vitality and wellbeing.

This book shows the importance of cellular health, the functions o the cells and what you can do to improve your cellular health. The most important thing is to be conscious about your own cellular health using the information in this book and all other information that is freely available for everyone. What you do with it, it totally up to you.

About the author

Jos Struik (1960) studied Dutch and English language and Business Administration.

He has had a long career in IT and consultancy working for Cap Gemini in the Netherlands and being an entrepreneur in several companies since 1996.

In 2012 he started a healthcare company together with his wife Caroline. This homecare company became very successful and grew to 800 employees and almost 4000 clients in 2017. In 2018 Jos and Caroline sold this company to the largest homecare company in the Netherlands.

With his experience in healthcare and seeing around him what impact (bad) health can have on life, he started to get interested in the cause of many diseases and found the importance of cellular health.

In 2018 he started his new company Vitalityfuture. Vitalityfuture helps people to find new and revolutionary solutions and products that make and keep you healthy and strong. Vitalityfuture focuses on slowing down aging, reducing pain, lowering oxidative stress, prevention and strengthening the body and mind on a cellular level in a natural way.

Made in the USA
Monee, IL
02 September 2020